WHAT'S INSIDE ME?

My HEART

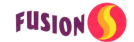
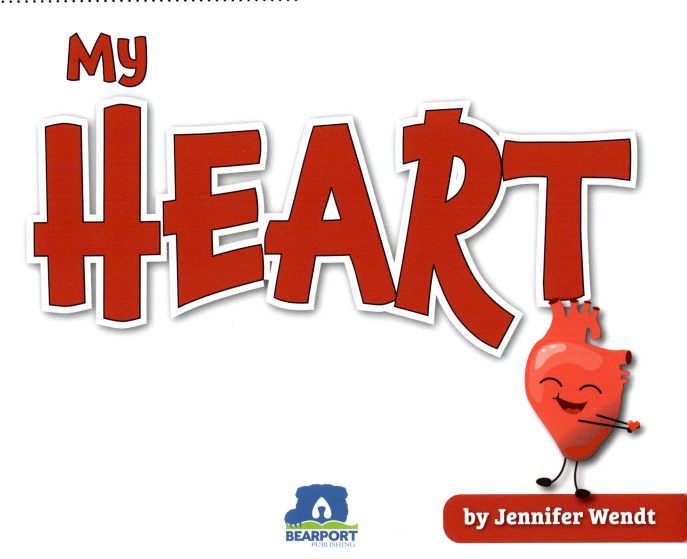

by Jennifer Wendt

BEARPORT PUBLISHING

Minneapolis, Minnesota

Credits: Cover, all background, © Piotr Urakau/Shutterstock, cover, 7, 23 © BlueRingMedia/Shutterstock, cover, 4, 10, 14, 16, 21, 22 heart illustration © Shutterstock; 4R Hurst Photo/Shutterstock; 5, 7, 9, 11–16, 18–19 (doodles) © Tiwat K/Shutterstock, 5 © LightField Studios/Shutterstock; 6 © Mopic/Shutterstock; 8L © Muhammad Fayyaz Rub/Shutterstock, 8R © Nixx Photography/Shutterstock; 9, 11 © Sedova Elena/Shutterstock; 12 © Pikovit/Shutterstock; 13 © The Faces/Shutterstock, 13 © studiovin/Shutterstock; 15 © S K Chavan/Shutterstock; 16 © innakreativ/Shutterstock; 17 © Christoph Burgstedt/Shutterstock; 18 © LightField Studios/Shutterstock, © Vera Vero/Shutterstock; 19 © Spotmatik Ltd/Shutterstock; 20 © Natalia Lisovskaya/Shutterstock; 21 © karelnoppe/Shutterstock.

President: Jen Jenson
Director of Product Development: Spencer Brinker
Senior Editor: Allison Juda
Associate Editor: Charly Haley
Designer: Oscar Norman

Library of Congress Cataloging-in-Publication Data

Names: Wendt, Jennifer, author.
Title: My heart / by Jennifer Wendt.
Description: Fusion books. | Minneapolis, Minnesota : Bearport Publishing Company, [2022] | Series: What's inside me? | Includes index.
Identifiers: LCCN 2021026722 (print) | LCCN 2021026723 (ebook) | ISBN 9781636914428 (library binding) | ISBN 9781636914497 (paperback) | ISBN 9781636914565 (ebook)
Subjects: LCSH: Heart--Juvenile literature. | Blood--Circulation--Juvenile literature. | Cardiovascular system--Juvenile literature.
Classification: LCC QP111.6 .W46 2022 (print) | LCC QP111.6 (ebook) | DDC 612.1/7--dc23
LC record available at https://lccn.loc.gov/2021026722
LC ebook record available at https://lccn.loc.gov/2021026723.

Copyright © 2022 Bearport Publishing Company. All rights reserved. No part of this publication may be reproduced in whole or in part, stored in any retrieval system, or transmitted in any form or by any means, electronic, mechanical, photocopying, recording, or otherwise, without written permission from the publisher.

For more information, write to Bearport Publishing, 5357 Penn Avenue South, Minneapolis, MN 55419. Printed in the United States of America.

CONTENTS

The Inside Scoop 4
Pumping Power 6
Heart Parts 8
The Value of Valves 10
Heart at Work 12
Heart Helpers 14
Keeping It Clean 16
Move for a Happy Heart 18
Eating for Health 20
Your Busy Body 22
Glossary 24
Index 24

THE INSIDE SCOOP

Your body is a super machine that keeps you moving, learning, and having fun. But how does it work? The secret is inside!

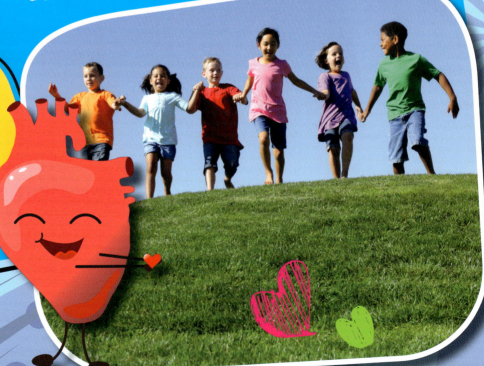

Show me some love by learning all about me!

When you run fast, you might feel a pounding in your chest. That's your heart working hard to help you play. Let's take a closer look.

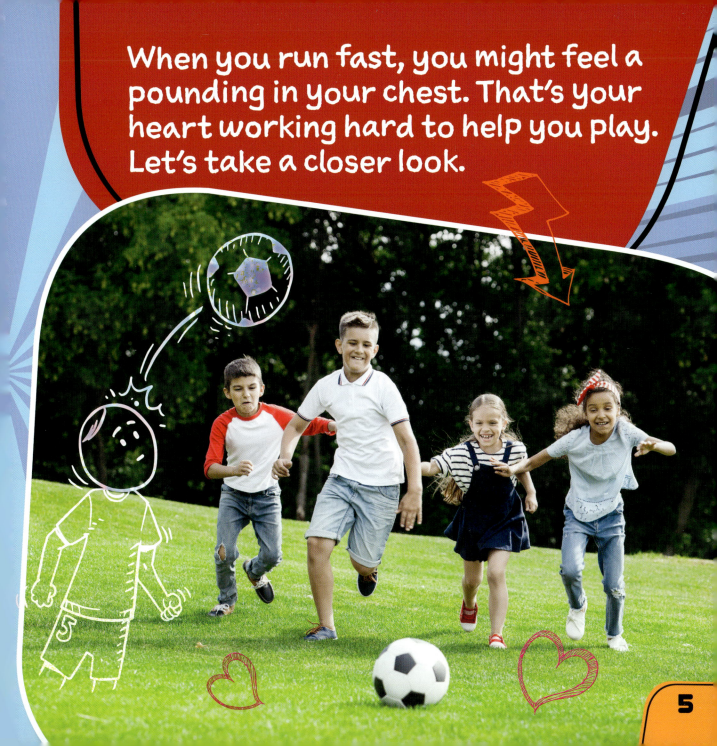

PUMPING POWER

THUMP-THUMP ... THUMP-THUMP!

Your heart is a **muscle** that pumps blood all over your body. It is pounding in the middle of your chest to keep you going.

Your heart beats about 70 to 115 times every minute!

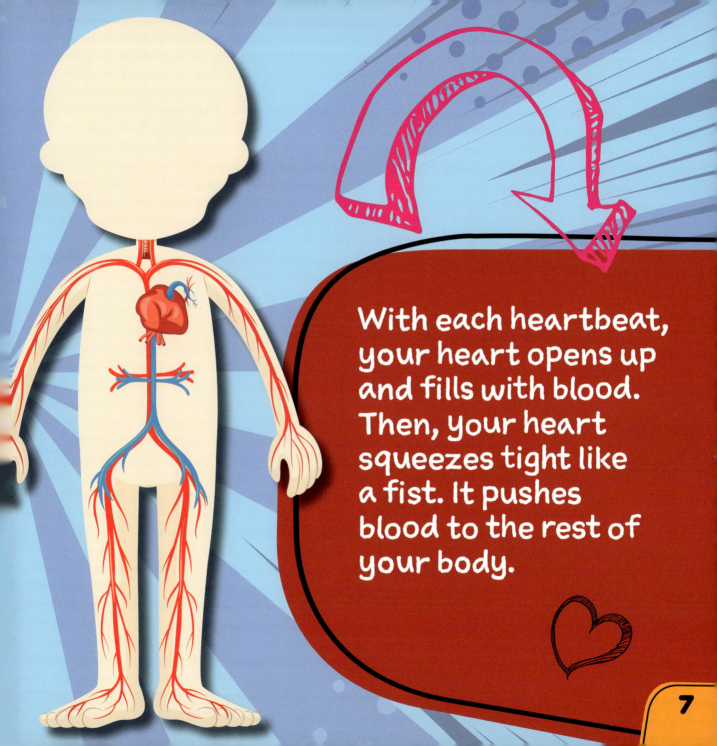

With each heartbeat, your heart opens up and fills with blood. Then, your heart squeezes tight like a fist. It pushes blood to the rest of your body.

HEART PARTS

The heart is made up of four different parts, called **chambers**. They split the heart from side to side and top to bottom.

An adult's heart is about the size of their fist.

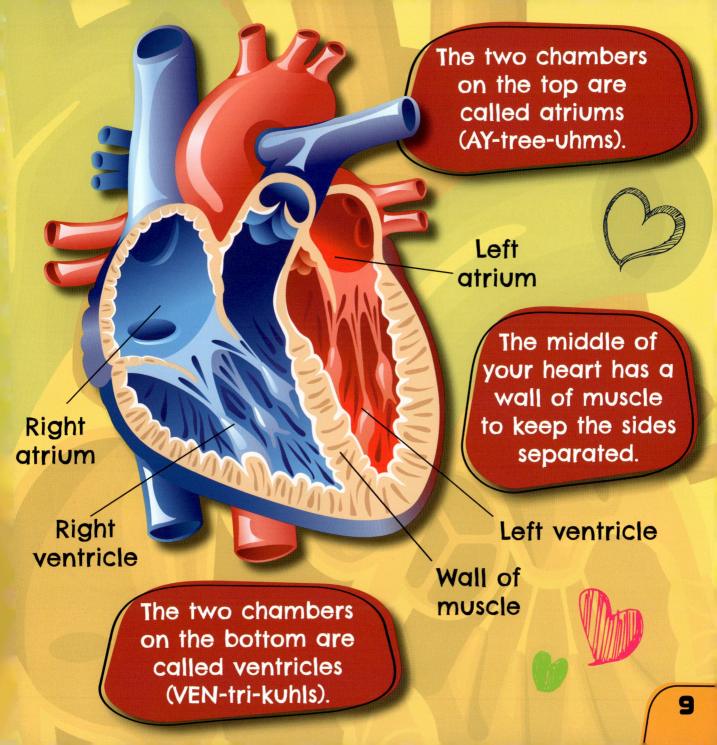

THE VALUE OF VALVES

Valves keep your blood flowing the right way. There are four valves in your heart. They open to let blood move forward. Then, they close to keep it from going back.

When I pump blood, valves help it go the right way!

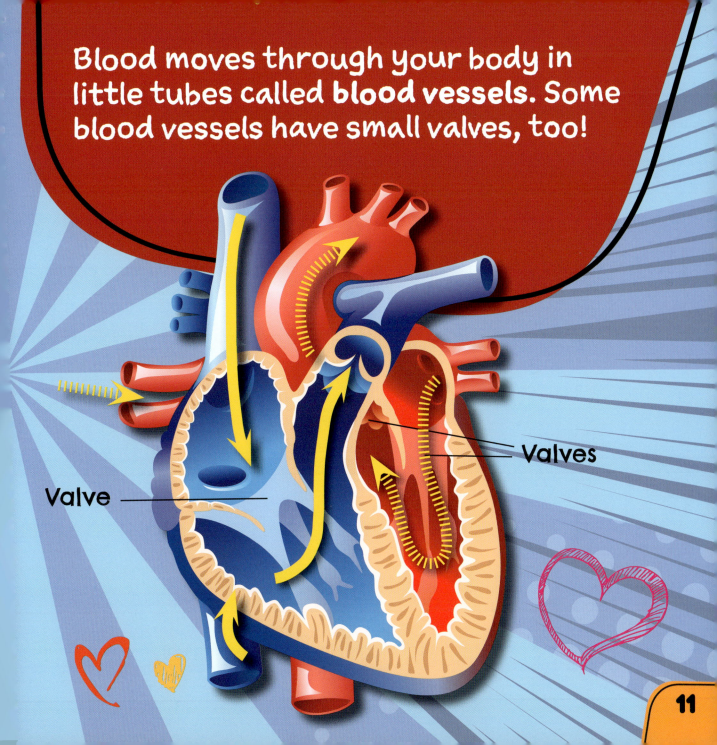

HEART AT WORK

Why does your *hard-working heart* need to keep your blood flowing? Because blood keeps you alive! It carries **oxygen** and other **nutrients** to all the parts of your body.

Blood moves through your whole body in less than a minute!

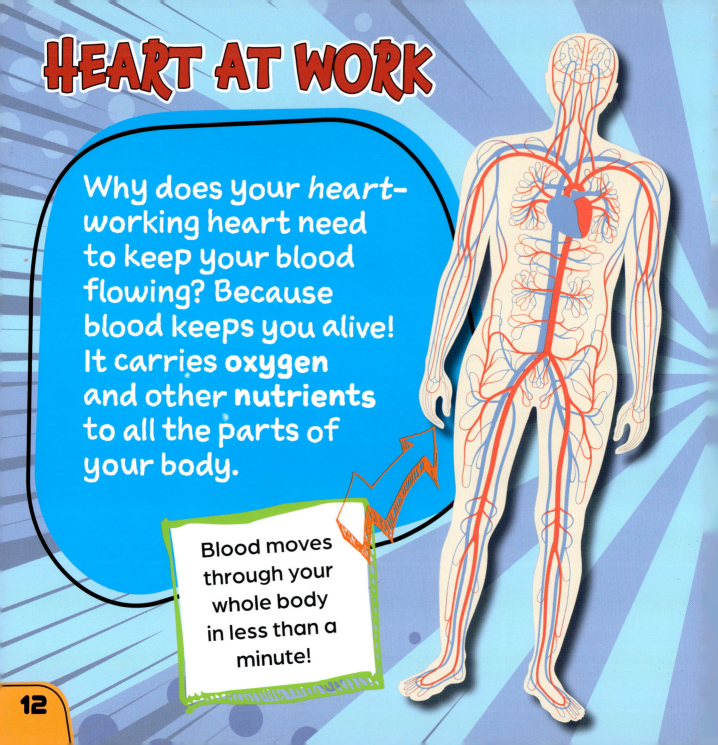

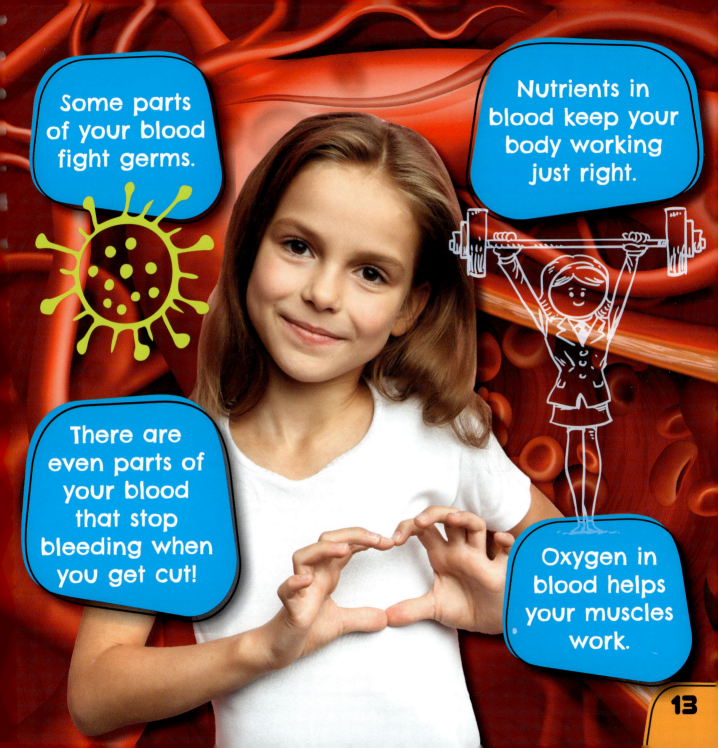

Heart Helpers

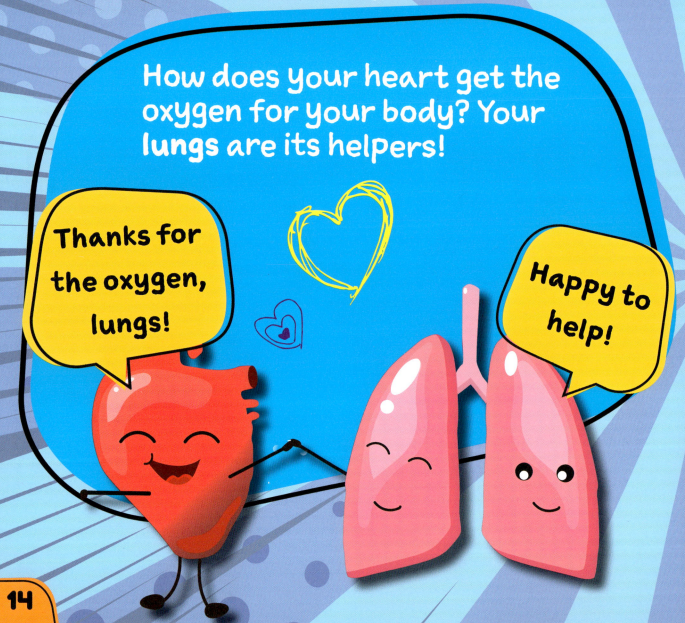

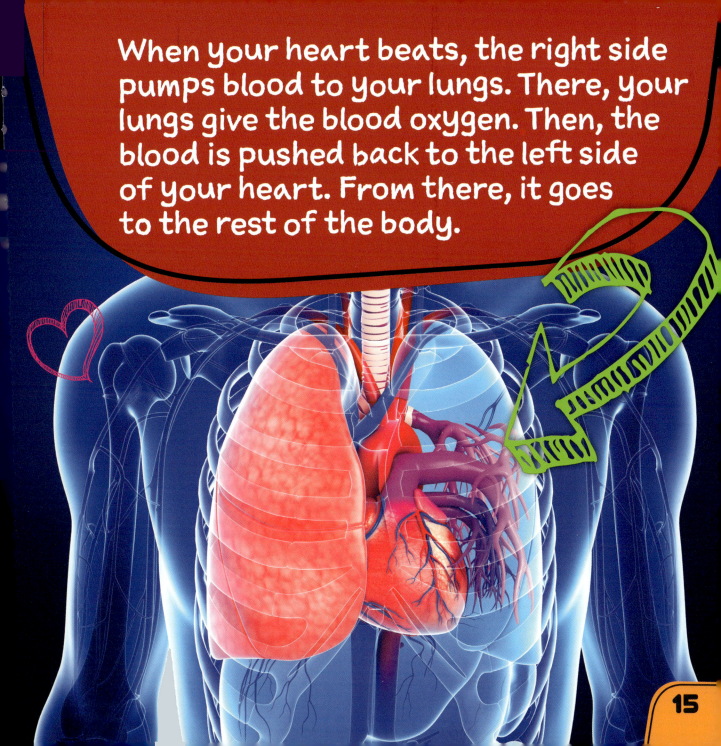

When your heart beats, the right side pumps blood to your lungs. There, your lungs give the blood oxygen. Then, the blood is pushed back to the left side of your heart. From there, it goes to the rest of the body.

KEEPING IT CLEAN

As blood travels through you, it picks up waste. Your pumping heart moves the blood to other parts of your body that get rid of the waste.

When I move your blood, it helps you take out the trash! You're welcome!

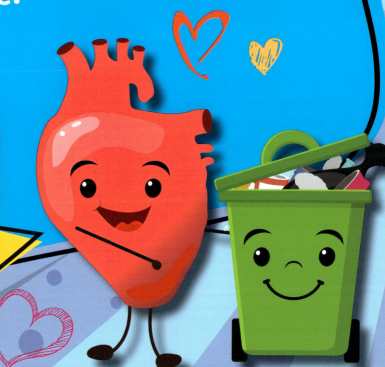

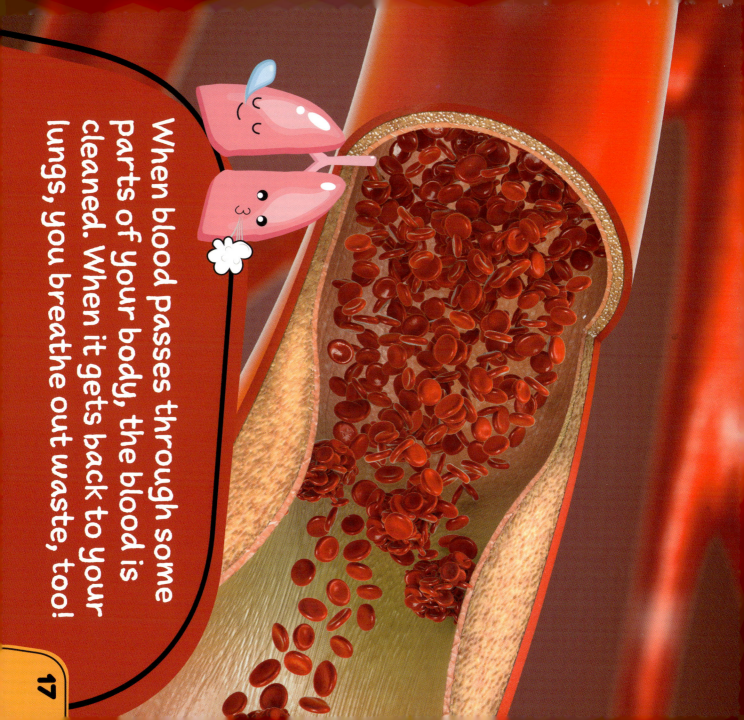

When blood passes through some parts of your body, the blood is cleaned. When it gets back to your lungs, you breathe out waste, too!

Move for a Happy Heart

Most people are born with healthy hearts. But it's up to you to help your heart stay that way. How can you keep your happy heart beating along? Exercise!

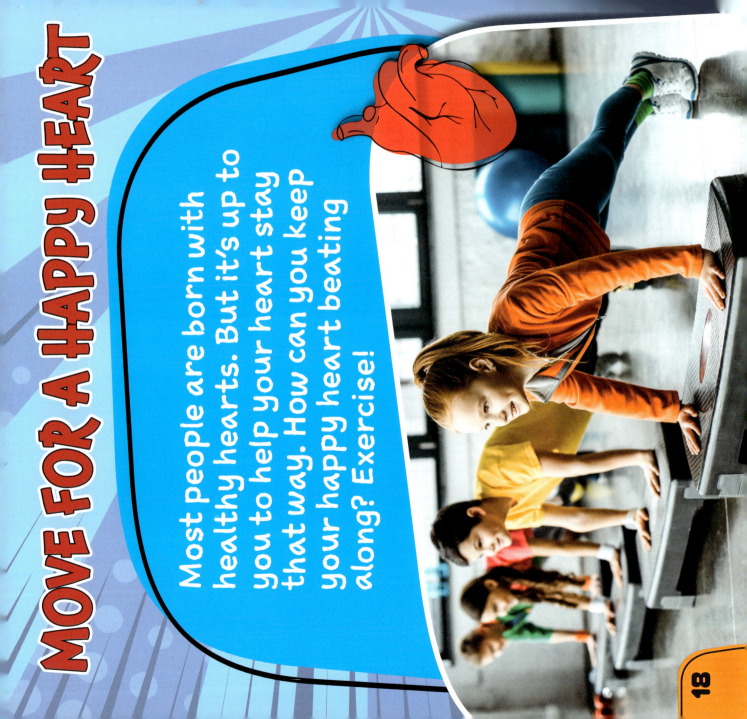

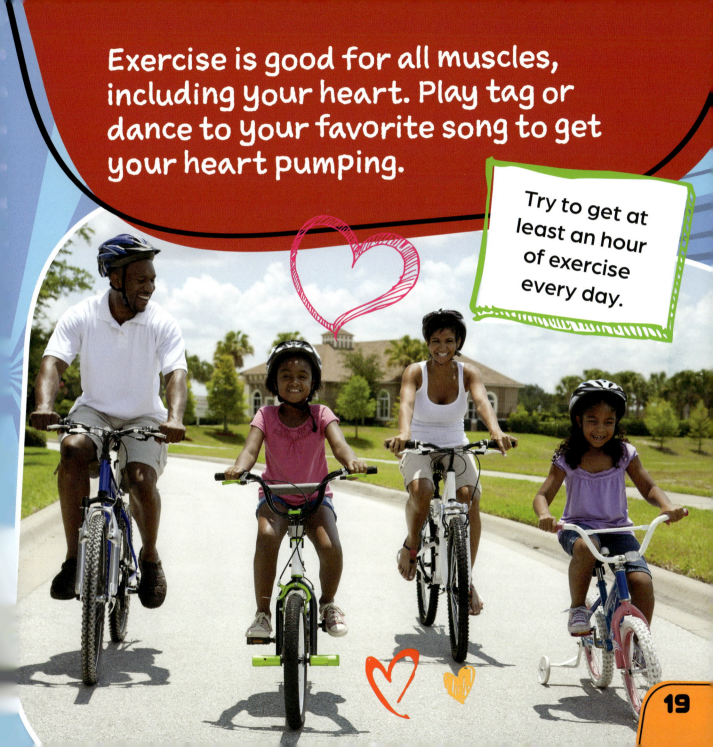

Exercise is good for all muscles, including your heart. Play tag or dance to your favorite song to get your heart pumping.

Try to get at least an hour of exercise every day.

EATING FOR HEALTH

Eating right is good for your heart, too. Get a mix of vegetables, fruits, and **whole grains** to keep your heart healthy.

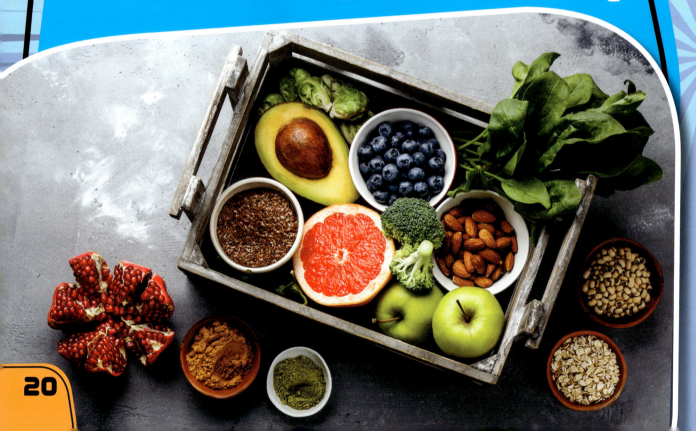

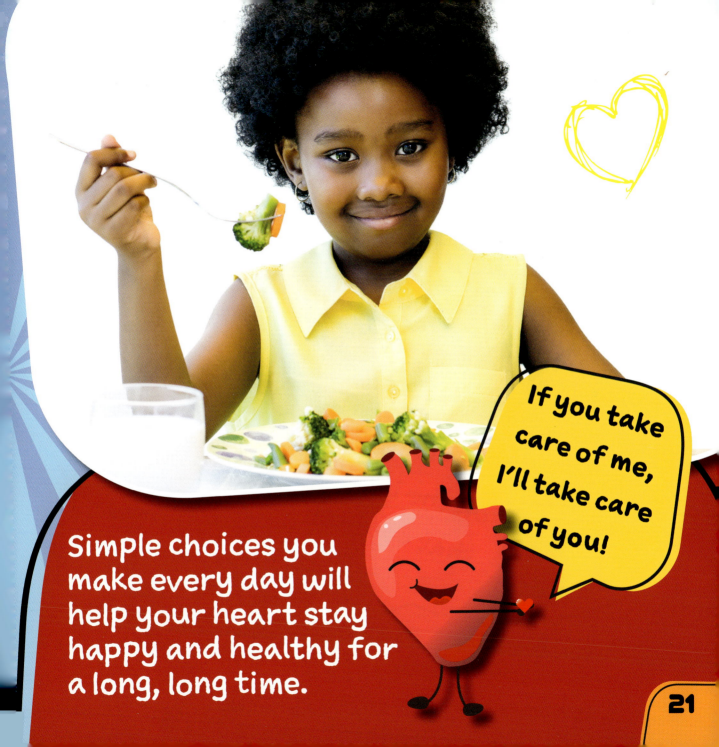

YOUR BUSY BODY

Your heart is an important part of the super machine that is your body. It works with lots of other things inside you. Together, they keep you going every day!

It's what's on the inside that counts!

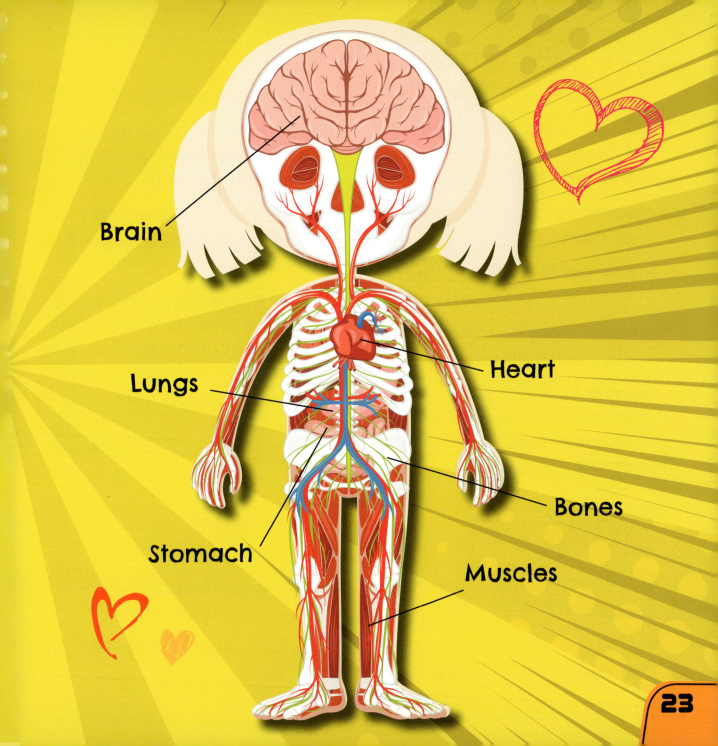

GLOSSARY

blood vessels tiny tubes that carry blood around a person's body

chambers closed-in spaces or parts

lungs parts of the body that are used for breathing

muscle a part of the body that helps you move

nutrients natural substances that plants and animals need to grow and stay healthy

oxygen an invisible gas in the air that people need to breathe to stay alive

valves parts of the body that control the flow of blood

whole grains the seeds of plants such as wheat that are kept whole and used as food

INDEX

blood vessels 11
chambers 8–9
eating 20
exercise 18–19
heartbeat 6–7, 15, 18
lungs 14–15, 17, 23
muscle 6, 9, 13, 19, 23
nutrients 12–13
oxygen 12–15
valves 10–11
waste 16–17